Pregna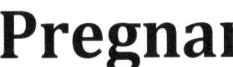

Everything an Expecting Mother Needs about Childbirth and Motherhood

Disclaimer

No part of this publication may be reproduced or transmitted in any form or by any means, mechanical or electronic, including photocopying or recording, or by any information storage and retrieval system, or transmitted by email without permission in writing from the publisher.

While all attempts and efforts have been made to verify the information held within this publication, neither the author nor the publisher assumes any responsibility for errors, omissions, or opposing interpretations of the content herein.

This book is for entertainment purposes only. The views expressed are those of the author alone, and should not be taken as expert instruction or commands. The reader of this book is responsible for his or her own actions when it comes to reading the book.

Adherence to all applicable laws and regulations, including international, federal, state, and local governing professional licensing, business practices, advertising, and all other aspects of doing business in the US, Canada, or any other jurisdiction is the sole responsibility of the purchaser or reader.

Neither the author nor the publisher assumes any responsibility or liability whatsoever on the behalf of the purchaser or reader of these materials.

Any received slight of any individual or organization is purely unintentional.

Tyler Backhause Copyright © 2015

All rights reserved. No part of this book may be reproduced in any form without permission in writing from the author. Reviewers may quote brief passages in reviews.

Introduction

I want to thank you and congratulate you for purchasing the book *Pregnancy: Everything an Expecting Mother Needs to Know about Childbirth and Motherhood.*

This book contains reliable and authoritative information to help you cope with the pregnancy situation intelligently and competently. This book is broken down into two parts: the first part is intended to help you have a real understanding of pregnancy and to teach you the appropriate measure to take in case you experience discomfort associated with your pregnancy. The second part provides you with detailed guidance on how you should take care of your newborn baby.

A pregnant woman experiences a sense of fulfillment and a special kind of joy. At the same time, there is natural anxiety and apprehension about the forthcoming confinement. The best remedy for this fear and anxiety is a complete understanding of pregnancy and childbirth. This knowledge and understanding can be obtained in one area, which is why it is wise to seek information from a health care provider or from informational books dealing with the subject in a comprehensible way.

It is necessary to understand what takes place during pregnancy and the measures to take in case of discomfort. A woman with this understanding will respond to various situations with insight rather than worry. The diverse and contradictory advice from friends, the report of various associated discomfort, and accounts of ordeals undergone by others in a similar condition makes the first pregnancy a frightening experience for a woman.

Reliable and authoritative information acquired beforehand can equip her to cope with the situation intelligently and competently and to overcome the needless fright. It is with this aim that this book has been written.

Thanks again for purchasing this book. I hope that you enjoy it!

PART 1
Chapter 1: Early and Late Signs and Symptoms of Pregnancy

Pregnancy signs and symptoms differ from woman to woman; you may experience some or none of the symptoms discussed in this chapter. One of the most common signs of pregnancy among women is delayed or missed periods. It is important to know the various signs and symptoms of pregnancy because each of them could either be related to a health condition or possibly to something other than pregnancy. This should be kept in mind while reading this chapter, and you should always consult your doctor if you suspect that you may be pregnant.

Within 6-12 days after conception, the zygote implants itself into the walls of the uterus. The zygote is the cell that is formed when two reproductive cells (the sperm and the egg) fuse together. During this particular period, you may start experiencing cramping and spotting. Some women do not ever experience this. Bear in mind that cramping or spotting is not by itself an immediate indicator of pregnancy and that it could simply be your regular menstruation cycle or some other type of health condition. You could still possibly be pregnant even if you do not experience any of these signs or symptoms.

A missed or delayed period is one of the earliest signs of pregnancy. When you become pregnant, you will automatically miss the next period post conception. Some women could potentially experience bleeding even after becoming pregnant. That being said, this sort of bleeding is shorter than the normal monthly period you typically would experience.

Your breasts become tender and enlarge in both size and fullness 1-2 weeks after conception. You may not notice this development of your breasts, but your breasts may become soft when touched or appear larger to other people who see them.

The feelings of tiredness and fatigue are also some of the early symptoms of pregnancy. You may start experiencing fatigue or tiredness as early as the first week after conception. Stress, depression, common colds, exhaustion, or other illnesses can also make you feel fatigued or tired; therefore, do not immediately interpret any fatigue or tiredness as a sign of being pregnant.

You may also start to experience morning sickness, which may start to show up 2-8 weeks after conception. With morning sickness, you may also start to vomit or feel nauseous during your pregnancy period.

You may also start getting headaches as well as lower backaches during the early stages of your pregnancy. However, you may also get a dull backache at any later stage of pregnancy. Backaches come as a result of impending menstruation, back problems, stress, or mental strains. You may also experience frequent headaches that occur because of dehydration, impending menstruation, caffeine withdrawal, eye strain, or other unidentified ailments.

At around 6-8 weeks after conception, you may also experience frequent urination or urine leakage. These problems most often occur as a result of temporary bladder control problems.
When you become pregnant, the skin around your nipples will also likely start to darken. This happens because of hormonal imbalances as a result of pregnancy. Hormonal imbalances are often the cause of various bodily and emotional changes at the beginning and throughout your pregnancy.

Your pregnancy may also cause cravings for certain foods. These cravings can last throughout your entire pregnancy although some women never experience this.

Chapter 2: What to Expect at your Prenatal Visits

Once you realize you are pregnant, you should schedule your first of many prenatal visits with your gynecologist. Get to know your doctor well because you will be seeing a lot of him or her throughout your pregnancy. Over the next nine months, you should expect anywhere between ten and fifteen appointments (and that's for a normal, low-risk pregnancy). Before calling to schedule your first appointment, be sure you know when your last regular period was. This will be a large factor in determining your due date.

Most doctors will schedule your first prenatal visit at around eight weeks after conception unless there are any pre-existing medical conditions that need to be addressed. If at this point you are taking any sort of medications, do not wait for your first visit to ask your doctor whether or not your medications are safe. Go ahead and ask whether or not you should stop taking your medications.

Your first prenatal visit tends to be the longest visit unless you experience any sort of medical problems along the way. At your first visit, you doctor is going to want to know all about your medical history. Make sure you are prepared to discuss any problems you have had in the past. Talk to your doctor if you mother or other close relatives had a difficult time with their pregnancies or labor. Your doctor will ask about your family history involving genetic and birth defects and will also explain your options for genetic testing.

Most practitioners will do an ultra sound at your first visit, but this is not always true. In addition to an ultra sound you can expect a thorough physical, a pap smear to check for cervical cancer, and a culture to check for certain STD's. Your doctor will also most likely ask for a urine sample, test for your blood type, and check for various other diseases that could make your pregnancy more difficult.

Your doctor is there to counsel you and to give you an idea of what is up ahead. Feel free to ask questions, and have your doctor address any concerns that you might have.

During your second trimester prenatal visits you will typically see your doctor every four weeks or so. During these visits your doctor will inform you of any test results from previous visits, ask questions about any concerns that arouse at previous visits, and ask you certain questions such as whether or not you have been feeling your baby move (and how often), whether or not you have been feeling nausea, if you have felt any contractions, have had any vaginal bleeding, and how your emotional state is. Your doctor will record your weight to be sure you are gaining at an appropriate speed. He or she will also check your urine for infections, check your blood pressure, and oftentimes he or she will want a blood test as well. Towards the end of your second trimester, your doctor will also test you for gestational diabetes; this test involves you drinking a sugar-filled drink (provided by your doctor) followed by a blood test. Gestational diabetes is common in pregnant women, so you definitely should expect this test towards the end of your second trimester.

Your third trimester visits start around your 28th week of pregnancy. You will begin seeing your doctor weekly rather than the ever four week visits. Your doctor will ask how you are feeling (emotionally and physically), ask about whether or not you have felt any contractions, and ask whether or not you have any concerns. Never be afraid to ask your doctor about any symptoms you have been having. You will experience various physical exams, be asked about your baby's movements, and possibly have your cervix checked on occasion to see if you have begun dilating. You can also request that your doctor check your cervix if he or she does not initiate the check.

Your doctor will likely check to see if you baby has "dropped" once you reach your due date. This is checking to see whether or not your baby has worked his or her way towards the pelvis in preparation for birth.

If your due date has come and gone, do not panic. Only 5% of women actually give birth on their due date. Some come early, some later. Your doctor will likely recommend you wait before scheduling an induction to see if you will deliver naturally. Most doctors will not allow you to go two weeks past your due date because of increased risks associating with late pregnancies. So do not worry- the longest you will likely go is the 42 week marker.

Try not to insist on scheduling an early induction because of worries or fear. Consult your doctor to determine whether or not you should induce.

Chapter 3: Foods to Eat When Pregnant

Proper nutrition during pregnancy is absolutely essential for your baby's growth and development. You should consume at least 300 additional calories daily than what you did before you became pregnant. This should include foods that are rich in all of the essential nutrients for your body as well as for your baby's health and physical development. The recommended daily requirements include 2 servings of fruit, 11 servings of grains and bread, 4 servings of dairy products, 4 servings of vegetables, and 3 servings of proteins (eggs, chicken, fish, meats, or nuts). You should consume sweets and fats sparingly as they can be (in excessive amounts) unhealthy for both you and for your baby.

You should eat foods that contain fiber such as cereal, rice, pasta, and whole-grain bread. You can also get your necessary fiber from most fruits and vegetables.

The foods that you consume daily should contain essential vitamins and minerals. If you think you are not getting enough of vitamins from your diet, you should supplement your body with a prenatal vitamin supplement. Regular use of these supplements will provide your body with the necessary vitamins that it needs. Always consult your healthcare professional before using vitamin or mineral supplements for taking the wrong ones could be unhealthy for your baby. Your doctor can prescribe a prenatal vitamin for you or advise you to purchase an over-the-counter brand that will help support your baby's growth and development and not be detrimental to his or her health.

During pregnancy you need to consume between 1000-3000 milligrams of calcium in your daily diet. You can get this amount of calcium by consuming at least four servings of dairy products and other calcium-rich foods each day. This additional calcium in your diet will greatly assist in your baby's bone development.

You should eat at least three servings of foods that are rich in iron such as spinach, breakfast cereals, beans, and lean meat. Iron is essential in the creating of hemoglobin, a protein found in red blood cells that carries oxygen to other cells throughout your body. This includes the traverse of oxygen to your baby. Make sure that your diet or dietary supplements are giving you up to 27 mg of iron daily. The use of any iron-rich supplements need to be approved by your doctor.

When you are pregnant, iodine helps your baby's brain and nervous system to develop. New studies suggest that an increase in iodine in your diet during pregnancy could greatly affect your baby's intelligence; iodine is also known to be a cancer preventative. You should make sure that you are consuming at least 250 micrograms of iodine daily. A variety of dairy products such as cheese, milk, and yogurt contain a sufficient amount of iodine. Cold navy beans, baked potatoes, and a variety of seafood such as shrimp, cod, or salmon can supplement your iodine requirements.

Your diet should contain at least 70 milligrams of vitamin C each day. There are plenty of benefits to vitamin C consumption including bone growth and repair, tissue repair, assisting the body with iron absorption, and it acts as an antioxidant to protect your body's cells from damage. You can get enough vitamin C from the daily consumption of oranges, strawberries, grapefruit, papaya, honeydew, Brussel sprouts, cauliflower, tomatoes, and mustard greens.

Once you become pregnant you will need at least 0.4 milligrams of folic acid per day. Folic acid deficiency could potentially lead to neural tube defects in baby. It can prevent certain birth defects surrounding your baby's brain and spinal cord development. These sort of birth defects can occur as early as 3-4 weeks of pregnancy, so it is essential that you start taking these sort of supplements early on. Choose foods that can give you enough folic acid daily. These foods include legumes (beans and peas), leaves, and dark green, leafy vegetables.

Choose foods that have sufficient amounts of Vitamin A. Vitamin A is important for the development of your baby's heart, lungs, kidneys, eyes, and bones. This vitamin is excellent at boosting infection resistance in your baby. It also helps with the circulatory, respiratory, and central nervous systems. Foods such as pumpkin, spinach, sweet potatoes, water squash, beet greens, turnip greens, carrots, and cantaloupe are all excellent sources of Vitamin A.

Chapter 4: Foods to Avoid When Pregnant

Avoid drinking alcohol and other addictive beverages during pregnancy. Alcohol consumption is linked to low-birth-weight, birth defects, mental retardation, and premature delivery. Fetal Alcohol Syndrome is also a serious birth defect that can be incredibly detrimental to your child, so avoiding alcohol during all stages of pregnancy is of the utmost importance.

The body doesn't require a large amount of caffeine. Never exceed the required daily amount of caffeine which is 300 mg/day while you are pregnant. Your baby's metabolism is still maturing, so it cannot fully metabolize large doses of caffeine. Because caffeine is a stimulant, it can greatly increase your heart rate and your blood pressure- neither of which is good for your baby. The quantity of caffeine in various drinks varies depending on the type of leaves and beans used and how it is prepared. One cup of black tea contains around 80 milligrams of caffeine while coffee contains about 150 milligrams. A 12-ounce glass of caffeinated soda contains around 30-60 milligrams of caffeine. You should also avoid dark chocolate since it contains a significant amount of caffeine.

Consumption of saccharin is not recommended during pregnancy. This substance passes through the placenta and gets deposited in the fetal tissues. Only use artificial sweeteners that have been approved by the FDA, such as sucralose (Splenda), acesulfame-K (Sunett) and aspartame (Equal or NutraSweet); these artificial sweeteners are considered safe. Always consult with your health care provider before the use of any of the above mentioned sweeteners.

The intake of foods that contain a large amount of fat is strongly discouraged. Monounsaturated fats and polyunsatured are the "good" fats that should make up the majority of the fats that you intake during pregnancy. Saturated fats, hydrogenated, and partially hydrogenated fats are the types of fats you should avoid. The recommended amount of fat during pregnancy should be only 30% of your total daily calories. If you are eating around 2000 calories a day, your total daily amount of fat should be 65 milligrams or less.

Cholesterol is associated with several medical conditions. During pregnancy high cholesterol can lead to pregnancy-induced hypertension. You should, therefore, limit your daily cholesterol intake to 300 milligrams, although dangerously low cholesterol can lead to premature labor and low birth weight if it is not kept in check.

Several types of seafood and fish contain mercury that is not good for the health of you and your baby. High levels of mercury can damage lungs, kidneys, and your baby's nervous systems. Mercury can also cause hearing and vision problems for your baby. Therefore, do not eat king mackerel, swordfish, shark, or tilefish. You should also avoid eating raw fish (clams and oysters).

Avoid consumption of soft cheeses such as Brie, feta, Camembert, Mexican-style cheese, and blue-veined. These cheeses are not pasteurized and may lead to a Listeria infection. Only eat yogurt, processed cheese, hard cheese, cottage cheese, or cream cheese.

Chapter 5: Dealing with Body Changes and Discomfort during Pregnancy

During pregnancy, you may be faced with several bodily changes and various forms of discomfort. You may feel sick and lose your appetite or find it increasingly difficult to keep certain foods down.

The uterus will continue to expand in capacity causing some pain and aches in the knees, feet, abdomen, thighs, pelvic bone, or groin area. This condition is called sciatica, and it is believed to occur when the uterus presses into the sciatic nerve. To deal with this problem, lie down and rest. You should also apply some heat in the affected areas. Call your medical care professional if the pain persists. Towards the end of your pregnancy, pelvic pain could also be caused by your baby "dropping" down into the birth canal. There are certain yoga and stretching positions you can try to assist with the later pregnancy pains; consult your doctor or midwife about safe positions you can try in an attempt to alleviate some of these pains.

A few months after conception, your breasts start to increase in size and fullness. As the delivery date approaches, you will experience rapid hormonal changes that may cause your breasts to grow even larger. In the third trimester, your breasts may start to leak colostrums. Wear a maternity bra to support your breasts and upper abdomen. You may also place nursing pads in your bra to absorb colostrums that may leak. Talk to your doctor if you discharge fluids other than colostrums. You should also see your medical care provider if you feel that your nipples change dramatically as this can be a sign of something other than hormonal imbalances caused by your pregnancy.

During pregnancy you may experience frequent constipation with the signs being dry stools and painful or infrequent bowel movements. Constipation during pregnancy is caused by higher levels of hormones in the body which slows down the rate of digestion. Higher levels of hormones also relax the muscles in the digestive system. These factors plus the pressure put on the uterus are what causes frequent and sometimes painful constipation. To deal with this problem, always drink 8-10 glasses of water daily and avoid consuming drinks that contain caffeine. You should also try to consume plenty of foods that have a significant amount of fiber such as fruits and vegetables. You should also do mild physical activity.

The pressure created by the growing uterus as well as hormonal changes during pregnancy often time causes heartburn and indigestion. The hormones greatly affect the digestive system's muscles. As a result, the peristalsis process is slowed down. Peristalsis is a series of wave-like muscle contractions that moves your food to various processing stations within your digestive track; when this process is slowed down, a number of symptoms such as heartburn and indigestion can occur. Pregnancy hormones also relax the valve that separates the stomach from the esophagus- allowing acidic food to flow back into the esophagus. This causes the feeling of heartburn, which could continue to get worse as the baby grows. To deal with indigestion or heartburn, eat small meals slowly several times a day instead of the common three large meals. You should also drink fluids between meals and do not eat fried or greasy foods. Avoid eating spicy foods and also avoid drinking citrus juice. Try not to go to bed right after meals. Consult your doctor if the symptoms fail to improve.

Hormonal changes during the first trimester can also cause extreme nausea and vomiting. This condition is often described as *morning sickness*. To deal with this problem, eat small meals slowly several times a day instead of the common three large meals. Avoid smells that may upset your stomach. Consume dry cereals, saltines, or dry toast before getting out of bed in the morning. You should also eat bland foods that are easy to digest and that are low in fat such as rice, cereals, and bananas. Sip clear, soft drinks, weak tea, or water when you start experiencing the problem. Ice water is beneficial to some women who are experiencing nausea. The sudden shock to your taste buds from ice cold water can sometimes subdue your nausea; you can also try sour candies. You can also try sea bands, a medical wrist bracelet that apply pressure points to certain nerves in your wrists; sea bands are most commonly used to cure sea sickness, but like many women you may find that it helps to curve your morning sickness as well.

You may start to experience stretch marks and skin changes during pregnancy. They most often appear on the abdomen, thighs, and breasts. They are caused by the stretching of your skin during the second half of your pregnancy. Your nipples may also turn darker during pregnancy. You may also develop a dark line on the skin that runs from the pubic hairline up to the belly button. Unusual moles or dark skin patches can also appear, but it is always a good idea to have these sort of skin abnormalities checked by your doctor even if they are a typical symptom of pregnancy because moles or sudden changes in skin tone can also be a sign of cancer. Some women experience what is known as the "pregnancy mask" which is a darkening of the skin around the eyes and nose that sometimes gives off the appearance of a masquerade mask; this typically goes away shortly after delivery. Normally, most stretch marks and other skin changes disappear after delivery while other skin changes can sometimes stick around for several months. Certain skin alterations caused by pregnancy may need a little extra help from a dermatologist to help get your skin back to normal, but most women's bodies tend to take care of moderate stretch marks and darkening patches on its own.

You may also experience frequent urination or urine leakage during pregnancy. These problems occur as a result of temporary bladder control problems. Your unborn baby exerts pressure on the pelvic floor muscles, urethra and, bladder causing frequent urination and urine leakage. You should take frequent bathroom breaks while pregnant. You should still drink plenty of water to curb dehydration and should not deny yourself of water simply to prevent excessive bathroom breaks. You can also do regular Kegel exercises to tone the pelvic muscles. If you experience burning during urination, know that it is probably an infection and you should consult your doctor immediately.

Hemorrhoids are a condition that causes pain, itching, and bleeding in the rectum. They are caused by blood vessels in the rectal area that have become swollen This condition is common during pregnancy, and it improves after delivery. It is most common during the third trimester, and they can also appear during delivery in the midst of the second stage of labor due to pushing. You should drink plenty of fluids to avoid dehydration- another major cause of hemorrhoids. It is recommended that you eat foods that are high in fiber such as fruits and vegetables. Never try to overstrain with bowel movements. If the pain gets worse, consult your health care provider. Your health care provider may recommend that you use witch hazel to soothe the hemorrhoids.

Chapter 6: Benefits of Exercise during Pregnancy

Regular exercise throughout your pregnancy can help you to stay healthy and fit, and it can greatly reduce a number of symptoms associated with pregnancy. Exercise can decrease backaches and fatigue associated with pregnancy, and improve your posture. Scientific studies also indicate that regular physical activity can help relieve stress, prevent gestational diabetes, and build more stamina needed for a safe and less painful delivery. If you were physically active before conception, you should continue with moderate exercises once you become pregnant.

If you are a career athlete, you should be monitored closely by your obstetrician once you become pregnant. If you have never done regular exercises before, you should consult your health care provider to recommend an appropriate exercise program for you once you become pregnant. Do not attempt strenuous activities that could harm the baby. Walking is considered safe if you have never done any serious training before. Swimming is also a gentler form of exercise that is no too strenuous.

Exercise may not be advisable if you have a medical problem such as diabetes, asthma, or any type of heart disease. You should not do any exercise if you have a low placenta, bleeding, spotting, history of premature births, weak cervix, or recent miscarriage. Consult your physician to recommend an appropriate exercise program for you. Your doctor can also recommend personal training guidelines depending on your medical condition. Be sure to take precaution during any sort of aerobic exercises if you have any sort of pre-existing condition such as anemia, obesity or underweight, orthopedic related issues, seizures, smoking, or any other health conditions.

During pregnancy, most exercises are safe to perform as long as you do them moderately with great caution. Physical activities such as swimming, indoor stationary cycling, brisk walking, low-impact aerobics, and elliptical machines are recommended. These activities benefit your entire body, have little risks for injury, and can be continued until birth. Racquetball and tennis are also safe activities, but they often bring changes in balance if you are pregnant. If you were doing moderate jogging before pregnancy, you could continue once you become pregnant. Involve yourself in activities and exercises that do not require any coordination or balance.

Chapter 7: Understanding Your Pregnancy Exercise Program

Certain activities and exercises can be harmful if performed during pregnancy. Avoid holding your breath when performing any exercise or activity for this will limit your oxygen intake. Never involve yourself in activities where falling is likely to occur. Such activities include horseback riding and skiing. Do not participate in contact sports such as football, softball, volleyball, or basketball. Avoid any exercise or activity that may cause even mild abdominal trauma and activities that require extensive hopping, jumping, skipping, running, or bouncing. When pregnant, avoid straight-leg toe touches, double leg raises, full sit-ups, and deep knee bends. Bouncing while stretching and waist twist movements while standing are also exercises that you should avoid during pregnancy. Finally, avoid performing exercises in hot, humid weather.

For maximum health and fitness, a pregnancy exercise program should condition and strengthen your muscles. Always start with warming up for 5 minutes and stretching for 5 minutes. Incorporate into your program at least 15 minutes of cardiovascular activity. You should be sure to measure your heart rate regularly throughout your workout routine. Cardiovascular activity should be followed by any aerobic activity with 5 to 10 minutes of gradually slower exercises that end with gentle stretching as a wind down activity.

Before you begin your exercise, wear loose fitting clothes and make sure that your breasts are supported by a good bra with excellent support. Wear shoes that are designed for the type of exercise you are going to perform to protect you from possible injuries. Perform your exercises on a flat, level surface to minimize exercise related accidents. Consume enough calories to meet the needs of your exercise program and pregnancy. Relax for a little while before you begin your exercises. Drink plenty of water before, during, and after your workout routine. Never exercise to the point of exhaustion.

You should keep in mind certain changes in your body when conducting your exercises. Always remember that your internal changes and developing baby require more oxygen and energy. Pregnancy hormones cause the joint and ligaments to stretch, increasing the risk of injury by making your muscles *stretchy* and more likely to tear. The extra weight and the uneven distribution of your weight during pregnancy shift your center of gravity. The extra weight also puts more pressure on your muscles and joints in the pelvic area and lower back, making it easier for you to lose your balance and fall.

Stop exercising if you feel chest pain, a headache, pelvic pain, abdominal pain, persistent contractions, or notice an absence or decrease in fetal movement and see your doctor immediately. Also see your doctor if you feel cold, dizzy, nauseous, or light-headed during or after any sort of physical strain due to exercise. Call your physician if you experience vaginal bleeding, abnormal vaginal discharge, irregular or rapid heartbeat, muscle weakness, or difficulty in breathing or walking.

Chapter 8: How to Plan for Childbirth in Order to Have a Successful Experience and Outcome

There are some things to consider when planning to give birth. Your first decision is to consider the health care provider who is going to assist you during delivery. You have many options on who will take care of you when pregnant, during delivery, and during the first few weeks after childbirth. When you choose your health care provider, you will need to consider whether your pregnancy is low-risk or high-risk. You will also need to consider your thoughts on natural deliveries and pain medications as well as your role in the overall decision-making.

You need to begin by formulating a birth plan along the side of your health care provider at least one month before delivery. A birth plan is a written document that integrates your childbirth wishes with what your health care provider thinks is practical. A birth plan is important because it helps to minimize the conflicts that may arise between you and your health care provider regarding your childbirth options.

When formulating your birth plan, consider the following factors:
- Is your pregnancy low-risk or high-risk?
- If your pregnancy is low risk, should you deliver at a hospital or at home?
- Do you want to give birth naturally, or do you want to receive pain medication?
- If you want to receive pain medication, what sort of medications would you like to consider taking?
- Is your husband/father of your child going to help you through the delivery, or would you prefer that your relative or friend help you?
- Do you know the signs of real labor, false labor, and premature labor?
- What are your thoughts on fetal monitoring, labor induction, and episiotomy?
- If you had a caesarean delivery previously, do you want to attempt vaginal delivery this time around?

If your pregnancy is considered low-risk, you may want to consider whether or not to deliver at the hospital or to take your chances and deliver at home. Home birth is considered safe and reasonable if your pregnancy is low-risk and you want to experience the natural feeling of giving birth. If your pregnancy is considered to be high risk, you should experience your labor and childbirth in a hospital. In the case of any pregnancy complication, there will be trained personnel and appropriate facilities to assist you in delivering safely. If you choose to do a home birth, considering hiring a doula or midwife who can assist you.

The more informed and prepared you are about pregnancy and childbirth, the more confident you will feel about your pregnancy and the birthing process. If you are informed and confident about your ability to go about childbirth, you will experience less pain and have a good childbirth experience. Childbirth is a natural experience with an excellent chance of a successful outcome. Even if labor and delivery fail to go exactly as planned, you should have confidence in yourself and your health care provider that your newborn baby will grow up to be happy and healthy.

Chapter 9: Understanding the Signs of Labor in Order to Know When to Proceed to the Hospital

Many women experience false labor and rush to the hospital only to be sent back home to wait for additional weeks or another month. Others fail to know exactly when they became pregnant and plan to wait for a long time, only to end up having an unplanned delivery at home or in the car. You should, therefore, know what signs to look for when childbirth is near. Understanding these signs will help you to know when to proceed to the hospital or when to call your healthcare provider.

A few days before labor, your uterus is ready and prepared for labor. Your cervix begins to ripen and soften. Your body may go through a number of changes. Your body starts to lighten up when the baby starts to push down into the pelvis. You will begin to experience pressure in the rectum and pelvis, pain and craps in the groin, or feel persistent backache. You may experience the sudden spurt of energy or possibly experience fatigue. The vaginal discharge will become thick, and sometimes you will begin to have diarrhea. Your vagina will likely then start to release a small amount of blood-streaked mucus.

Sometimes you may experience false labor and feel the need to rush to the hospital. If you have irregular contractions that are not frequent or that do not get worse over time, you should know that it is not yet time to give birth. You should know that you are most likely experiencing false labor when the contractions are short in duration or low in intensity. During false labor, the pain is normally confined to the groin or lower abdomen rather than the lower back. When you experience these contractions, you will know that your cervix and uterus are now prepared for labor. You should, therefore, monitor the contractions to see if they are intensifying or becoming more frequent. If you are uncertain as to whether or not you are in false labor or actual labor, try changing positions. If you are standing, sit. If you are sitting stand up or lie down. You could also try going for a short walk to see if the contractions stop. If the contractions continue, call your healthcare provider to help you determine whether or not a hospital visit is necessary.

Proceed to your hospital or call your health care provider if you experience regular contractions that are increasing in frequency and intensity or if the pain is worse than you anticipated. You should also call your health care provider if you feel a trickle or gush of clear fluid flowing from your vagina. This shows that your fetal membranes have ruptured and that delivery is near. Call your healthcare provider if you are not sure whether you are in labor or not.

PART 2
Chapter 10: Taking Care of Your Newborn Baby at Birth

Your baby is finally out of the womb. At birth, the baby may look different from what you expected. Their skin typically appears mottled and vernix-a white waxy substance covers them. If your baby is crying, he or she may turn red from head to foot. During cold conditions, the feet and hands may turn blue. Do not worry if you notice these changes. Within 48 hours, your baby's skin color will become normal. Regardless of the condition of the child, you will need to take care of it.

Immediately after birth, you should pat the skin of your newborn baby dry to minimize heat loss caused by the evaporation of amniotic fluid from the skin. You should also wipe off the blood, vernix, or stool from the skin to keep the baby clean. Usually, the remaining vernix on the skin will be absorbed after 48 hours.

Before birth, the mother's body regulates the temperature of the baby. After birth, the baby needs to maintain his or her body temperature. You should, therefore, keep your baby warm by wrapping him or her with a soft blanket. Make sure to monitor the baby's temperature. You can also keep the baby in skin-to-skin contact with your body. This is another way to ensure that the baby's temperature is stable. Skin-to-skin is now known to help your baby in greater ways than what was known previously; if you are unable to participate in skin-to-skin with your newborn due to delivery complications (such as having a cesarean) you can encourage your baby's father to snuggle up with baby chest to chest just as you would. Skin-to-skin, in addition to health benefits for your baby, is also a wonderful bonding exercise that can help your baby grow more attached to his or her mother and father as well as stabilizing his or temperature. You should not bathe your newborn baby until their temperature stabilizes.

Studies indicate that some sexually transmitted diseases like gonorrhea and Chlamydia can be transmitted from mother to baby during vaginal birth. These conditions are known to cause eye problems in newborn babies. You should, therefore, give your baby erythromycin (antibiotic eye ointment) within two hours after birth if you have any of these STDs. This antibiotic prevents eye infection that may be caused by these diseases. Do not use eye drops on your baby until you consult your doctor.

At birth, your baby has a temporary shortage of certain vitamins. Your newborn baby needs vitamin K to ensure the proper clotting of their blood. Your baby should, therefore, get a vitamin K injection within the first few hours of birth. Normally, the injection is given into your baby's thigh muscle but can also be administered orally in a series of doses when breastfeeding.

Hepatitis B is a virus that infects the liver. This virus can be passed from the mother to the baby during the first few months of birth. If your baby is infected at birth, it will develop chronic hepatitis B. Your baby should, therefore, be immunized against this virus shortly after birth. If you were infected with hepatitis B during pregnancy, your baby should be administered with the hepatitis B immunoglobulin drug and hepatitis B vaccine immediately after birth.

Immediately after birth, your baby's umbilical cord is clamped and cut. You should remove the clamp after 48 hours. The stump of the umbilical cord on your baby's navel is moist and looks bluish-white at first. However, after some time, it will quickly lose water and become black and dry. There is no need to dress the stump. It will dry itself if it is exposed to air. Over time the stump will fall off on its own.

Within the first few days after birth, your baby should pass greenish-black, tarry stool known as meconium. You should, therefore, monitor your baby to ensure that this happens. Once you start breastfeeding your child, the stool will turn to a seedy yellow-green. Make sure there is no delay in stool passage. If there is any sort of delay, it may be a sign of disease. Your newborn baby should urinate at least once every 24 hours. Once you start to breastfeed your baby, urination should occur approximately four to five times every 24 hours.

About two-thirds of newborn babies develop jaundice. Jaundice is a condition where the baby's skin and eyes turn slightly yellow in color. This happens when there is too much build-up of the chemical bilirubin in the baby's body. Normally the liver or the bowel system is responsible for the removal of this substance from the body. The liver of the newborn baby may not be mature enough to remove this chemical, leading to building up of this chemical in the body. If your newborn baby shows signs of jaundice, you should monitor his bilirubin levels. Your health care provider may recommend a heel-prick blood test. Very high levels of bilirubin may cause deafness or brain damage, so it is important to monitor this. Your doctor may then prescribe phototherapy for your baby to help dissolve the yellowish pigment from his skin.

Chapter 11: Getting to Know the Behavior of Your Newborn Baby

When your baby is born, he or she comes into this world capable of doing many things. Your baby is capable of listening to sounds, cooing and gurgling, and trying to orient his head towards voices. Your baby is able to imitate your facial expressions and also move his arms when excited. Even though a newborn baby's vision is limited, they enjoy looking at faces. Your baby can detect shadows, light, contours, shapes and movements.

Your face has certain features that can capture your baby's attention. Always talk, nod your head, or smile when looking at your newborn baby. If your baby is enjoying this kind of interaction, he will continue looking at you. If the baby feels that he is not interested in you, he may look away. Do not feel rejected or unwanted when the baby looks away. This is a normal part of your baby's development. When your baby looks away, let him look away.

Some signals can be more difficult to detect than others. You should be patient with yourself to study and learn the baby's signals that tell you how he or she is feeling and how you should react. When your baby cries, it is a sure way of telling you that something is wrong with him or her. Your baby may be feeling distressed or uncomfortable. You should, therefore, comfort your baby when he or she cries. As your baby continues to grow, he or she will learn from your comforting that you care for him or her. Your baby will have confidence that you will be there in case of any distressful or uncomfortable situation.

Your newborn baby sleeps about 18 hours each day. However, of these sleeping hours, he only spends about 20% in a deep sleep. The rest of the time, your baby will drift in and out of sleep. This means that by the time you put him down to take a nap, he or she will likely be awake and crying. This can be exhausting, but if you breastfeed him for a longer amount of time, he will sleep for longer hours.

Your newborn baby also spends a considerable amount of time feeding. For the first few weeks after birth, your baby will feed when he is hungry. Your baby should be breastfed at least eight times per day. Each breastfeeding session should last between 5 to 10 minutes. A healthy baby should pass bowels at least every 3 to 4 hours a day in the first few weeks. This means you will be doing a lot of diaper changing each day.

Your baby may spend his hours in a quiet state, or your baby may spend much of his or her time crying. His little lungs are capable of wailing for a long time, and this can become overwhelming at times. Always keep in mind that crying is the only way that your baby can communicate with you. As he continues to grow and develops other ways of communication, his crying will decrease.

Chapter 12: Safety Measures You Should Take to Ensure That Your Newborn Baby Is Safe

Your newborn baby is not as weak as you may think. However, you still need to handle him or her with care to keep him or her safe and secure. When you hold your newborn baby with your hands, make sure that you support his or her head with one hand. Although your baby's body is strong, his or her head will remain fragile for the first few months after birth.

You should purchase a child car seat that meets federal standards. Whether the safety seat you have purchased is new or used, make sure that it is installed properly. Your newborn baby may not like to be fastened in the car seat at first, but with time he or she will get used to it. If you have never installed a car seat before, you can have the installation checked at your local police station or hospital to insure your child's safety.

Make sure that all of the other equipment for your newborn baby, including cribs, carriers, strollers, bassinets, playpens, changing tables, and toys, meet national standards. If you purchase secondhand equipment, also meet the national safety standards. You should also ensure that this equipment is kept clean all the time to prevent your baby from becoming sick.

Babies like to cry all the time when they feel distressed or uncomfortable. Because of tiredness or frustration, you may be tempted to shake or hurt them. Never attempt to do this because shaking your baby may damage his or her brain. If you feel like shaking your baby or hurting him or her, get help instead from your relative, friend, parent, or healthcare professional. If you do not have immediate help on hand, set your baby down in his or her crib and walk away until you calm down.

You should always feed your newborn baby with warm foods. You should never heat your baby's bottle in a microwave. The bottle may be warm to touch, but the content inside may turn out much hotter than expected. If you still have to use a microwave, check the temperature of the bottle and its content before giving it to your baby.

Babies like rolling or turning when placed in stationary areas. They also like rolling or turning when their diapers are wet or soiled. To prevent your newborn baby from falling when placed in open areas, always put one hand on him all the time. Be exceptionally careful if you put your baby somewhere up high; do not remove your hand or your baby could roll over and fall.

Never leave your newborn baby in the care of a child, locked in a room alone, or in a bathtub. Your child may drown in the bathtub if left unsupervised. Use a small tub to bathe your newborn baby to minimize the chances of him drowning in it. Always check the temperature of the bathwater before putting your baby in it. Never allow your babysitter to bathe your newborn baby.

Do not leave your newborn baby alone with a pet. Keep emergency phone numbers ready just in case there is an accident involving your child at home. You may consider taking a child safety awareness class so that you will know what to do in case there is an emergency.

Newborn babies are prone to sudden infant death syndrome (SIDS). You can reduce the risk of your child getting this disease by placing your baby on his back to sleep. Do not put your newborn baby to sleep on his tummy since this position is considered a prone position for suffocation. Once your baby is at an age in which he or she is able to roll over onto his or her stomach and back again with ease, the changes of sudden infant death syndrome drop significantly. Also, ensure that the any puffy blankets or pillows allow your newborn baby to breath comfortably. It is recommended that you avoid using pillows at all.

Chapter 13: Mother's Milk-Baby's Ideal Food

Breast milk is best for your newborn baby because its benefits extend beyond basic nutrition. The breast milk contains all of the nutrients and vitamins that your baby needs for the first six months. It also contains antibodies that protect your newborn baby from illness. Studies have also found that breastfeeding is good for your health as well.

In a nutshell, breastfeeding protects your newborn baby from several illnesses. Studies indicate that respiratory illnesses, stomach viruses, meningitis, and ear infections occur less often in breastfed babies, and they are less severe when they do occur. Studies have also found that breastfeeding provides your baby with protection against illnesses throughout the remainder of their lives and not just in infancy. It can also reduce your baby's risk of developing certain childhood cancers. You should try has as much as possible to feed your baby exclusively breast milk. This means that they should be given no solid food, water, formula, or supplements for the first six months. Most doctors recommend trying to go at least the baby's first full year of life before attempting to wean.

Breastfeeding can protect your baby from developing allergies. If you give your baby soy milk or cow's milk, he or she will be more allergenic than if they could have been given breast milk. Scientists say that certain immune factors are only available in breast milk and can help prevent allergic reactions to various foods and other substances.

Studies also indicate that breast milk could boost your child's intelligence significantly. In a study of more than 20,000 infants studied from birth to 6 years, researchers found that there were improved cognitive abilities of babies who were fed exclusively on breast milk for the first six months after birth. Yet another study found that babies with extremely low birth weight who were breastfed shortly after birth improved their mental development scores and physical growth at two years. Babies that are born premature particularly can benefit from breast milk as well.

Breastfeeding may also protect your child from obesity. The American Academy of Pediatrics says that those infants who are fed exclusively on breast milk have less of a risk of becoming overweight. Experts also say that infants who are given breast milk are better at eating until their hunger is satisfied. It is also known that breast milk contains less insulin than other infant supplements and formulas. Additional studies have indicated that breastfed babies have more leptin in their bodies. It is a hormone that researchers say plays an important role in regulating fat and appetite.

Breastfeeding may lower your baby's risk of sudden infant death syndrome (SIDS). A study that was conducted in Germany and published in 2009 found that if you breastfeed your baby exclusively on milk for the first six months it will prevent SIDS.

Studies also indicate that breastfeeding can reduce your risk of postpartum depression and lower your stress level. It is also known that many women report a feeling of relaxation when they breastfeed. According to the research conducted by the National Institute of Health, it was found that women who stopped breastfeeding early or who did not breastfeed at all had a higher risk of developing postpartum depression.

Breastfeeding may reduce your risk of some types of cancer. Several studies have indicated that women who breastfeed are more protected against ovarian and breast cancers. For breast cancer, you should breastfeed your child for at least one year to have the most protective effect.

Chapter 14: Dealing With a Constantly Crying Baby

Crying is the first language that your newborn baby is using to communicate with you. If you soothe a crying baby and he stops crying, you will feel happy and relieved. But if you soothe a crying baby and he continues to cry, you likely will feel frustrated. You should, therefore, understand what to do or how to respond when your baby is crying.

During the first three months after birth, some babies cry more than others. All babies cry most during the early evening or late in the afternoon. Many studies have shown that the crying of babies follows a particular development pattern during the first three months of birth. This model is referred to as a crying curve. Crying starts to increase at 2 to 3 weeks after birth, peaks at around 6 to 8 weeks after birth, and gradually declines when the baby reaches 12 weeks of age.

Depending on the intensity of crying, you should be able to guess correctly what your newborn baby wants. At three months of age, your baby may use different cries to mean different things. If your baby is hungry, your baby may start crying quietly and slowly but continue to cry louder with rhythm. You should, therefore, feed your baby routinely to prevent him from crying.

Your baby may cry because of pain. The typical cry for a child with pain is high-pitched, harsh, tense, non-melodious, short, sharp, and loud. You should, therefore, look into what is hurting your baby to prevent him or her from crying.

If your child is upset, he or she may cry in an intermediate, mild way. This fussy cry differs from the hunger cry. However, both can sound the same. Fussy crying includes when your baby wants to be held or when a soiled diaper is causing discomfort. Sometimes your baby may cry because of frustration with lack of sleep.

A crying that is high-pitched and persistent and up to three times higher than the normal crying or a low-pitched cry that is persistent can be associated with some sort of chronic illness. These types of crying are different from the regular baby cries, and you should never confuse it with excessive crying that is identified as colic.

A child may also cry frequently and intensely a condition often referred to as colic. Your baby may cry three hours per day, three times per week, or at least three weeks consecutively. The excessive crying as a result of colic may begin in the second week after birth and continue toward the end of the second month. Your baby may intend to stretch out their legs and arms or draw in their feet and arms tightly to their bodies. His or her stomach may become swollen and tight. There is growing evidence that colic is associated with brain development and the digestive system. Colic normally disappears between three and four months of age, but it has been known to last up to a year. Colic does not cause any sort of long-term problems with the baby, but it can put detrimental amounts of stress on you and the family. If you have a baby with colic, know that it is only temporary and get as much support as you can from loved ones. Swaddling, gentle cuddling or swaying, and a pacifier can sometimes soothe a baby with colic at least temporarily.

Chapter 15: Health Issues in Your Newborn Baby

Your newborn baby may keep you on your toes. You may end up being frustrated on what to do if your baby suffers from infections, eye problems, fever, spitting up, behavior changes, vomiting, constipation, or diarrhea. Just remember that you are not alone; consult your doctor when necessary and rely on friends and family for help.

Your baby may be born with developmental problems in one or more of his organ systems. This is a common problem that affects about 3% of all births in the world.

Your baby may also have a chromosomal abnormality or have a genetically determined disorder. These health disorders may present challenges for you and for your newborn baby when he gets older, especially if they are left untreated. As a mother, you may have dreamed of a perfect child. You may feel disappointed when you realize that your newborn baby will be faced with these abnormalities. You need to consult your health care professional if you suspect any sort of developmental problem so that your baby can get immediate assistance. You may not realize that some forms of medical therapy and surgery can be very helpful in treating some of these defects.

Your baby may not have a clear, radiant skin like the ones that you see in TV commercials. To ease your worries, know that most of those babies on TV are probably wearing makeup to cover up their own skin abnormalities. You may deliver a baby with a number of skin conditions or birthmarks that some have historically associated with curses or witchcraft, but do not worry- your baby just has some unusual skin blemishes. Some of these skin conditions disappear a few years after birth. Others may remain throughout your child's lifetime. You have to consult your healthcare provider when you realize that your baby's skin condition is becoming a health concern.

Your newborn baby has a weak immune system. You should, therefore, ensure that your child is breastfed during the first six months of birth. Breast milk contains important antibodies that help fight your baby's infections and strengthen his immune system. If you exclusively breastfeed your baby during the first six months, your baby will have fewer infections. If infected by diseases, a breastfed baby also responds quickly to treatment. If you suspect that your newborn baby has an infection, take him to the doctor to start taking antibiotics immediately.

Spitting up breast milk or formula shortly after feeding is common among many newborn babies. Spit-up typically rolls out of the baby's mouth with a burp. You should differentiate spitting up from vomiting. Spitting up is less quick and less forceful than vomiting. Vomiting is often associated with stomach infections, gastrointestinal problems, or a reaction to something that a baby ate.

Diarrhea is common in newborn babies. This is when your newborn baby passes very runny, watery stool in more volume or at an increased frequency than normal. Diarrhea is often associated with vomiting, and it is caused by a viral or bacterial infection. Constipation is also common among newborn babies. This is a condition whereby the baby's bowel movements are hard and cause bleeding or pain. A constipated baby groans or strains when trying to pass stool.

Chapter 16: Growth and Development

Once your baby is here, you may start to wonder what is normal in term of his or her growth and development. Know that every baby is different and your baby being a little bit behind of the average is not something to cause alarm, but let's take a look at what you most likely can expect in your baby's first year of life.

In those first couples of weeks of life you will probably notice some fluctuation in your baby's weight. Do not panic; this is perfectly normal. When your baby is first weighed in after birth you will likely be surprised as how big your little baby is. This initial weigh in is known as the *birth weight*. Most of the time, your baby will lose a considerable amount of that birth weight within the first few days of life. Continue weekly pediatrician visits or check in's until your baby works back up to that initial birth weight to be sure that he or she is eating sufficiently and has not gotten sick.

As early as three weeks old your baby may start experiencing growth spurts. A lot of parents find that they are throwing out a considerable amount of newborn clothes with your baby outgrowing clothes before he or she even gets a chance to wear them! You will know that your baby is going through a growth spurt if he or she suddenly is wanting food more often and in greater quantity. For breastfeeding moms you probably have just now gotten to the point where your baby is not demanding food every hour or two, but suddenly he or she is back to suckling hourly. Do not worry- this demanding feeding schedule will only last a couple of days- until your baby's next growth spurt that is!

By six weeks old you may start noticing that your baby is finally getting on some sort of schedule. Its' okay if he or she is still a little inconsistent, but at this point you may want to start looking for advice from your doctor (or possibly family members) about how to get your baby on a more normal sleeping schedule. Do not worry if it takes a little longer for your baby though because every child is different.

By two months old your baby will likely be getting ready to start rolling over, reaching for toys, and maybe even sitting. By three months your baby will most definitely be on a more regular feeding and sleeping schedule. Most babies start teething around four months, but some will begin as early as three and others as late as twelve.

At six months your baby will start mastering what is known as the pincer grasp: grabbing small objects with the thumb and forefinger. Around seven months your baby will likely be clapping, pointing, and waving. A true personality is developing in your baby now. Most babies begin crawling around eight months, so if you have not already baby proofed your house now would be the time. By nine months your little crawler will become a climber! Be sure to keep a careful watch on your baby around stairs because he or she is going to want to climb them. Most babies will start walking anywhere between nine and eighteen months, so you may want to start shoe shopping fairly soon.

Again, keep in mind that every child is unique in terms of developmental milestones. If you are concerned whether or not your baby is behind, consult your doctor before you start to worry.

Conclusion

It is necessary to understand what takes place during pregnancy and why and also the measures to take in case of discomfort. A woman with this understanding will respond to various situations with insight rather than worry. The diverse and contradictory advice from friends, the report of various associated discomfort, and accounts of ordeals undergone by others in a similar condition makes the first pregnancy a frightening experience for many women. My hope is that this book has greatly helped you in some way or another.

Please do not be someone who just reads this information and does not apply it. The strategies in this book will only benefit you *if you use them*!

If you know of anyone else that could benefit from the information presented here, please let them know about this book.

Thank you, good luck, and congratulations on your new bundle of joy!

If you enjoyed this book, please feel free to leave an honest review. Also, check out some of my other popular raw food and vegan books listed below:

Easy Vegan Recipes for Children: A simple guide to vegan cooking that even your children will love.

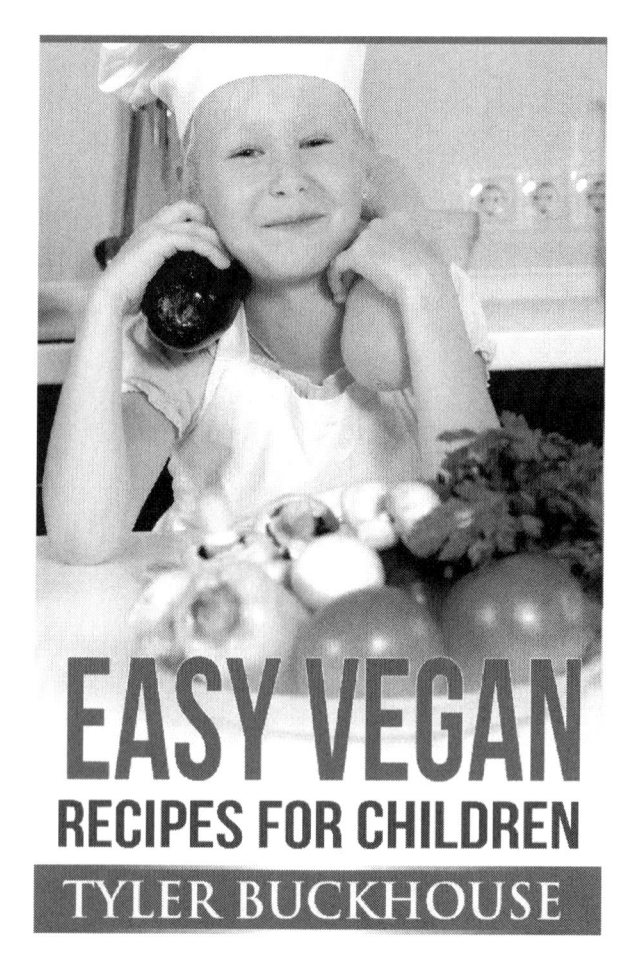

How to Lose Weight While Playing with Your Kids

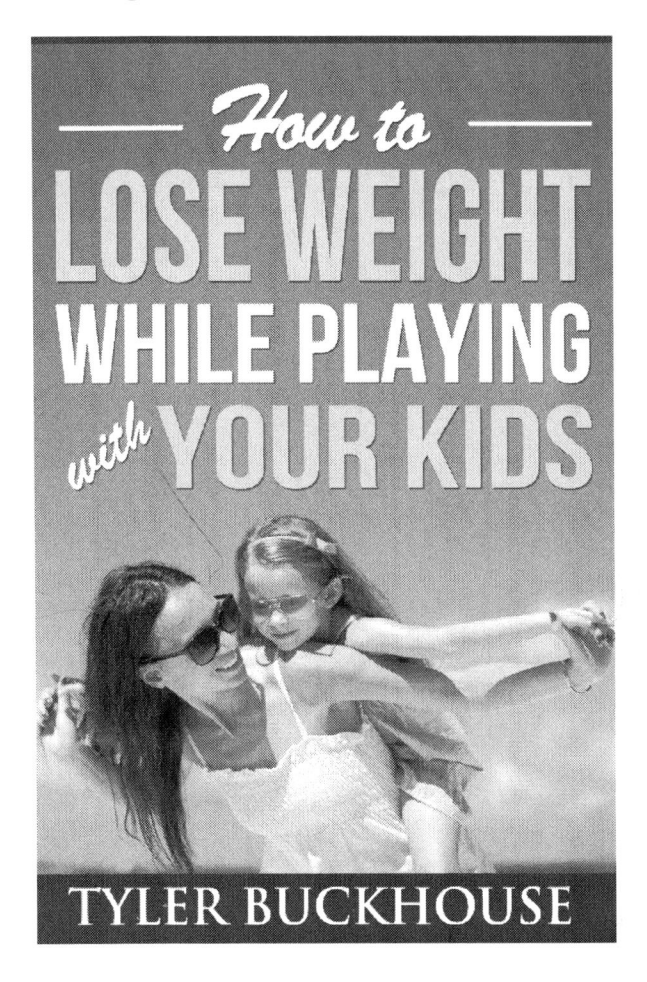

Printed in Great Britain
by Amazon